Better Life Diet©

TABLE OF CONTENTS

Foreword by Robert H. Knopp, MD............................... iv-v

Introduction -- Lester R. Sauvage, MD........................... vi

Section I:
Nutritional Basis for the
Better Life Diet and
Weight Control... 1-16

Section II:
Sample Seven Day Meal Plan and
Nutritional Analysis for the Better Life Diet............ 17-26

Section III:
Exercise - - Essential Ally of Diet 27-53

Section IV:
A Simple Plan for a
Long and Youthful Life....................................... 54-63

Section V:
Glossary.. 64-71*

Index 72-73

Special Notes 74

* This is not the usual glossary consisting of definitions. It is instead an easily understood series of mini-lectures of key subjects. You may find that reading through this glossary first gives you the broader insight needed to more readily apply the advice in the other sections.

Foreword by
Robert H. Knopp, MD
Professor of Medicine,
Director of the Northwest Lipid Research Clinic,
University of Washington

Interest in nutrition information has never been greater on the part of the general public. Scientific findings reach the media daily, often in advance of their appearance in the scientific literature and well in advance of the ability of dedicated scientists to consider and test the latest ideas for veracity.

How do we explain this appetite for information and what does it mean? My personal view is that changes in the American lifestyle, the lack of time to cook or even of families to eat together, the penetration of public consciousness with advertising to consume convenient and not necessarily nutritious food-stuffs have left us in a state of nutritional disorientation in the past approximately 40 years. It is no wonder that people are reaching out for help.

Consider the earlier situation. Typically women did the cooking. Skills were passed on to daughters who shared in the household responsibilities. Styles of cooking were governed by tradition and an agrarian history that favored preparation of a variety of homegrown fruits and vegetables, many of which were canned or frozen for winter. Sources of refined carbohydrates were fewer and were treats; highly sugared cereals didn't exist. Remember Shredded Wheat? By virtue of an agrarian or nearby agrarian tradition (like open air markets in cities) and without much premeditation, the right thing was being done for the most part with respect to fresh fruits, vegetables and unrefined carbohydrates.

Not everything was right about this dietary scenario, though. The diet was rich in saturated fat. Perhaps by working very hard at heavy farm work or industrial labor, there was much less obesity and a high saturated fat diet might have been tolerated. But adding in cigarette smoking, a phenomenon of the 20th century, is more than any heart can stand, leading to a heart disease epidemic. Dr. Sauvage has spent the greater part of his life combatting this epidemic with his surgical knife and his words of advice.

Where are we now? In our modern life, healthy traditions are even more tenuous. Men and women are both responsible for the work of the home, including nutritional choices. We rarely have heavy daily physical work as a justification for a high-fat diet or as an antidote to obesity. Meanwhile, we are deluged with TV ads to eat things we don't want and we don't even have to stand up to change the channel.

In the course of finding a new way to good eating, sound advice is needed that is understandable to men as well as women. The **Better Life Diet** espoused by Dr. Sauvage falls within the general boundaries of the sound nutritional advice offered by major national bodies. It studiously avoids extremism. It takes advantage of the fact that restriction of saturated and *trans* fatty acids and a reduction in fat intake overall can lead to a reduction in blood cholesterol and some weight loss. With Dr. Sauvage's recommended restriction of saturated and *trans* fatty acids to 10% or less of total calories, the fat intake from these threatening sources falls between the National Cholesterol Education Program Step I and Step II Diets. The **Better Life Diet** also avoids high intake of refined carbohydrate and the blood sugar surges that ensue while providing essential fiber, antioxidants and omega-3 fatty acids. The amount of protein that is recommended is greater than typically suggested but may aid satiety and spontaneous or intentional weight loss, in keeping with recent studies. The exercise recommended is very practical and is an essential adjunct to maintenance of normal weight and well-being.

Most importantly, the **Better Life Diet** is conceived and written with the intensity and directness of a leading heart surgeon who draws on the experience of repairing the ravages of advanced atherosclerosis and advising patients who know they are in trouble. In this age of fraying tradition, redistribution of responsibilities, media distraction and jobs that provide no exercise, the **Better Life Diet** offers direct no-nonsense, mainstream advice from a voice of great experience.

Introduction to Better Life Diet©

My objective is to help you live longer by enjoying the most healthy, yet satisfying, diet available, the **Better Life Diet**.

There are so many conflicting diets that the average person is left in a swirl of confusion. To mention a few -- the *Pritikin* and *Ornish* diets advise 80% of calories from carbohydrates, 10% from fats, and 10% from proteins. The popular *Atkins* diet advises next to no carbohydrates in the initial phase while encouraging unlimited quantities of fat and protein. The *Sugar Busters* diet avoids sugar. *The Omega Diet* focuses on types of fatty acids. The *American Heart Association* diet advises a high carbohydrate and moderately restricted fat intake. The *Protein Power* and *Zone* diets advocate high protein consumption.

I have selected the best from these diets and combined this information with what I have learned in taking care of thousands of people. As a surgeon my long-term goal has been to help people stay healthy and out of the operating room. This **is** the better way! The result is the **Better Life Diet** -- the diet for the vast majority of people. This is a diet for taste and long life.

I believe that most deaths from heart attacks, strokes, and limb loss; nearly all cases of lung cancer and emphysema; and a great many cases of adult-onset diabetes, blindness, and kidney failure can be prevented.

Sound impossible? Far from it. Here's a formula that will work for any of us: don't smoke, follow the **Better Life Diet,** exercise regularly, achieve and maintain a healthful weight, and control your psychological responses to life's challenges, *i.e.* stress. If you implement these rules for healthy living, your chances of living a long and youthful life overflowing with happiness will be greatly increased.   Sincerely,

Section I:
Nutritional Basis for
The *Better Life Diet* and *Weight Control**

There are three basic types of foods: **carbohydrates, fats,** and **proteins.** Carbohydrates and proteins are calorie poor (four calories/gram). Carbos provide energy, fiber, and vitamins. Proteins form enzymes, hormones, antibodies, building materials, muscles, and energy. Fats are calorie rich (nine calories/gram). Fats make cell walls, hormones, energy, insulation, and padding.

The **Standard American Diet ("S.A.D.") causes many to die prematurely.** It has too many calories, too many low-fiber carbohydrates (white bread, mashed potatoes, french fries, and white rice), far too much refined sugar, too much saturated fat, and too many *trans* fatty acids. In addition to their improper and excessive diet, most Americans don't exercise nearly enough.

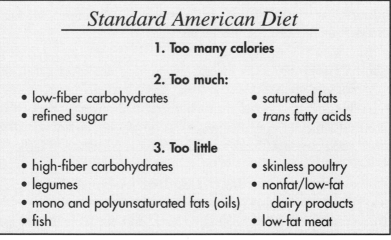

Figure 1 - Some deficiencies of the Standard American Diet.

* **We become what we eat. See glossary for discussion of carbohydrates, cholesterol, fats, fiber, insulin, proteins, refined, sugar, and *trans* fatty acids.**

1

More people are dieting. Yet more people are obese. Why? Too many diets fail to distinguish between high, low, and non-fiber (sugar) carbohydrates, saturated (bad) and unsaturated (good) fats, and high and low bad fat protein sources. Bad fats, *trans* fatty acids, and excesses of low-fiber carbohydrates and refined sugar (which are converted into saturated fat) decrease the liver's ability to remove LDL cholesterol (pp. 65-66) from the blood. High blood levels of this chemical cause heart attacks and strokes. To reduce LDL cholesterol one must exercise and avoid eating fatty meat, unskinned poultry, low-fiber carbohydrates, refined sugar, whole milk, cheeses made from whole milk, cream, butter, and foods made with them as pies, cakes, and ice cream, and commercially processed hydrogenated foods such as most margarines, crackers, cookies, candies, doughnuts, and desserts.

The average American eats 150 lbs of refined sugar/year, yielding 760 calories/day -- 38% of the calories in a 2,000 calorie diet. Sugar (sucrose) contains no fiber, minerals, phytochemicals, or vitamins -- only calories. Pop and watered-down juice drinks are full of sugar -- 10 teaspoons in a popular cola (ten times the total glucose in all the blood in your body).

For real people in the real world we advise our **Better Life Diet** that provides about **50%** of calories from carbohydrates, mainly from high-fiber varieties (very little refined sugar); about **30%** from fats, mainly "protective" or "good" types; and about **20%** from good proteins (those with little associated saturated fat).

We have designed the **Better Life Diet** for health and taste. A good diet makes eating a pleasure, not a punishment. See pp. 17-26 for examples of the healthy, tasty, and fulfilling meals the **Better Life Diet** will bring you. This diet is for long life and joy.

Most carbohydrate calories should come from high-fiber sources (fresh fruits, fresh vegetables, legumes, whole-grain breads, cereals, and pastas, and whole grains, such as brown rice). Fiber slows digestion of carbohydrates, minimizes fluctuations in blood sugar (glucose), and reduces appetite. **Few calories should come from low-fiber sources and fewer still from refined sugar.**

Most fat calories (20% or more of total) should come from oils, *i.e.* liquid (unsaturated) fats. Monounsaturated oils are good for us, such as olive, canola, avocado, and peanut. Some polyunsaturated oils are excellent, too, such as soybean, walnut, fish, and flaxseed. Calories from saturated fats and *trans* fatty acids, however, should not exceed 10% of the total. Saturated (hard) fats (as in butter) and hydrogenated oils (such as in many margarines) are soft solids at room temperature. Excesses of these "hard fats" are far worse for our arteries than is the cholesterol in an extra scrambled egg.

Most protein calories should come from fish (p. 10), skinless poultry (skin contains the bad fat), eggs, legumes, nuts, seeds, nonfat/low-fat dairy products, and low-fat meat such as lean beef, lamb, and center cut pork loin/chop or roast. Few protein calories should come from expensive cuts of red meat or from unskinned poultry because both have a high content of saturated fat.

This selective high-fiber carbohydrate, unsaturated fat (oil), and good protein *Better Life Diet* protects our arteries from hardening and clotting. This diet prevents the marked rises and falls in blood glucose and related insulin secretion that cause recurring waves of profound fatigue, uncontrollable hunger, and excessive eating throughout the day which leads to obesity, diabetes, and high blood pressure (hypertension) -- all powerful risk factors for coronary heart disease. (See p. 67 for omega-3 guidelines.)

The *Better Life Diet* combined with a good exercise program (pp. 27-53) is optimal for the vast majority of people who wish to look and feel their best. For the few whose livers can't remove LDL cholesterol from their blood (a "gene" problem, p. 63), we advise physician prescribed cholesterol-lowering medications in addition to the **Better Life Diet** and **Exercise Program**.

Foods High in Saturated Fats
and
Foods High in *Trans* Fatty Acids

Restrict calories from these sources to not more than 10% of total calories consumed daily.

Saturated Fats:
1. Fatty red meats (marbled) and unskinned poultry.
2. Canned meats.
3. Processed meats such as bacon, luncheon meats, and sausage.
4. Lard and foods made with lard.
5. Butter and foods made with butter.
6. Coconut, palm, and palm kernel oils, and foods made with these saturated tropical oils
7. Cream (sour/table/whipped), and foods made with cream, including rich ice creams.
8. Milk, whole or even reduced fat milk (p. 8), and foods made with them, such as high-fat cheeses.

Trans Fatty Acids:*
1. Margarines and foods made with them.
2. Commercially processed foods made with hydrogenated "oils"* such as crackers, cookies, cakes, candies, doughnuts, pies, and other pastries.

* Most types of margarines and many commercially processed foods (as listed) contain hydrogenated soybean or other oils. Hydrogenation changes these oils into soft solids at room temperature. This change occurs because hydrogen is added to the molecular structure of the oils, and this produces *trans* fatty acids. Unfortunately, these acids are as dangerous as saturated fats because they also impede the removal of LDL cholesterol from the blood by the liver. This effect of hydrogenation causes the LDL cholesterol levels to rise. Such elevations become dangerous when they reach 130 mg/dL (an average value) -- pp. 66-68,71.

Who doesn't look forward to sitting down with family and friends to enjoy a good meal? Though eating is pleasurable and necessary for life, we must control what we eat to live a long and healthy life. The **Better Life Diet** does this. This diet is based on seven broad goals. It does not depend on detailed calorie counting. Enjoy this diet for life. Use it to lose, maintain, or add weight as needed.

The Seven Goals of the Better Life Diet

To reduce obesity, adult-onset diabetes, blindness, kidney failure, cancer, hypertension, heart attacks, strokes, limb loss, aneurysms, and hemorrhages, we advise the following seven dietary goals:

1. **Eat plenty** of high-fiber carbohydrates such as fresh fruits -- an apple a day is hard to beat; fresh vegetables; legumes; whole-grain breads, cereals, and pastas; and whole grains, such as brown rice.
2. **Markedly restrict** low-fiber carbohydrates (white bread, mashed potatoes, french fries, and white rice).
3. **Drastically restrict refined sugar.**
4. **Choose** the protective monounsaturated oils, such as olive, canola*, and peanut; and polyunsaturated omega-3 oils (walnut, fish, and especially flaxseed).
5. **Severely restrict** saturated fats and *trans* fatty acids.
6. **Enjoy** low saturated fat protein foods -- fish, skinless poultry, eggs (p. 11), legumes, nuts, seeds, nonfat/low-fat dairy products, and low-fat meat, as lean beef, lamb, or center cut pork loin/chop or roast. (Shellfish OK.)
7. **Drink** at least two quarts of water a day (8 glasses).

   * also high in omega-3 fatty acids (p. 67)

If you are significantly overweight, this balanced **50-30-20** diet of high-fiber carbohydrates, protective fats, and good proteins, when combined with a suitable exercise program (pp. 27-53), will autoregulate your weight over weeks to months to where you will both feel and look your best and will enable you to stay that way.

Good Proteins - 20%

• Fish
• Skinless Poultry   **4 cal/gm**
• Eggs
• Legumes
• Nuts and Seeds
• Nonfat/low-fat Dairy
• Low-fat Meat

Protective Fats - 30%

       9 cal/gm

• 2/3 or more from mono and
   polyunsaturated oils (pp. 3,5)
• 1/3 or less from saturated fats and
   trans fatty acids (p. 4)

High-Fiber Carbohydrates - 50%

• Fresh Fruits   **4 cal/gm**
• Fresh Vegetables
• Legumes - - Peas, Beans, and Lentils
• Whole-Grain Breads, Cereals, and Pastas
• Whole Grains, such as Brown Rice,
   Wheat, Oats, Barley, and Bulgur

*Figure 2 - Building Block Diagram of the **Better Life Diet** reflects a calorie origin of 50% from carbohydrates (mainly high-fiber varieties), 30% from fats (mainly protective mono and omega-3 and -6 polyunsaturated types), and 20% from proteins (mainly those categories that have little association with saturated fats). Also see pages 9,10.*

The areas of the **Better Life Diet** Building Block Diagram accurately reflect the origin of calories from carbohydrates (50% - 4 cal/gm), fats (30% - 9 cal/gm), and proteins (20% - 4 cal/gm). For a 2,000 calorie daily intake, this means 250 grams of carbohydrates, 67 grams of fat, and 100 grams of protein.

The **Better Life Diet** emphasizes high-fiber carbohydrates, unsaturated fats (oils), and good proteins (Fig. 2, p. 6). While this diet doesn't eliminate any foods, it markedly restricts low-fiber carbohydrates (white bread, mashed potatoes, french fries, and white rice), drastically restricts refined sugar, and severely restricts saturated fats and *trans* fatty acids.

This tasty diet assures an adequate supply of calories (energy), building materials, fiber, minerals, phytochemicals, vitamins, and water. Also, the **Better Life Diet** markedly reduces the glucose (sugar) stimulus for excess insulin secretion which further protects against the development of obesity, adult-onset diabetes, and hardening of the arteries (atherosclerosis).

The **Better Life Diet** requires the use of nonfat or low-fat milk. There are four designations of milk according to its fat content: whole, reduced-fat, low-fat, and nonfat.

Whole milk contains too much saturated fat and so does reduced fat milk. A cup (8 ounces) of whole milk has 150 calories and 5 grams of saturated fat (4%); a cup of reduced-fat milk has 120 calories and 3 grams of saturated fat (2%); a cup of low-fat milk has 100 calories and 1.5 grams of saturated fat (1%); and a cup of nonfat milk has 80 calories and no fat. People who are lactose-intolerant can usually handle four ounces of milk or drink calcium-fortified soy milk at a meal.

The **Better Life Diet** provides 30% of total calories from fat, mainly from unsaturated fats (oils) that protect our arteries, such as olive, canola, nut, soybean, fish, and flaxseed oils. Even though these oils are good for us, they, like all fats, are so high in calories (9 calories/gram) that they must be taken in moderation. In addition, the calories from saturated fats and *trans* fatty acids should not exceed 10% of total calories. Also, the **Better Life Diet** requires a marked reduction in low-fiber carbohydrates and a drastic reduction in refined sugar (pp. 2,3 and below*).

* Sucrose (table sugar) is digested rapidly. This drives the blood glucose up which suppresses hunger and causes the pancreas to secrete insulin. Glucose falls. Hunger returns. When more sugar is eaten, the cycle repeats. Fats and proteins have little effect on insulin. Vegetables (because of their high fiber content) and fruits (because of their fiber and type of sugar -- fructose) convert more slowly into glucose and stimulate less insulin secretion. Milk sugar (lactose) causes a lesser insulin response, too. Insulin enables all the cells of the body to use glucose for energy, causes glucose to be stored as glycogen (p. 65), converts excess glucose into saturated fat when the limited glycogen stores are filled (p. 14), and prevents fat from being used for energy.

The up-and-down sugar-insulin relation fans the appetite; fats and proteins suppress it. Eating sugar throughout the day increases the secretion of insulin and enhances the manufacture of saturated fat from glucose, thereby negating the benefit of reducing the intake of saturated fat in the diet. But, markedly restricting low-fiber carbohydrates and drastically restricting refined sugar in the diet lowers insulin secretion and enables fat to be used for energy when the glycogen stores are exhausted. Making this source of energy available serves to help correct obesity and to prevent adult-onset diabetes, blindness, kidney failure, and hardening of the arteries.

The Better Life Diet all but deletes table sugar, standard soft drinks (soda), sugary "juice" drinks with less than 50% "fruit juice", jams, jellies, candies, cakes, pies, other pastries, ice creams, and most other desserts. By following the Better Life Diet, the average daily consumption of refined sugar in a 2,000 calorie diet can be easily reduced from about 760 calories to 120 calories (pp. 17-26).

People with fat around their waists have a significantly greater risk of high blood pressure, diabetes, early heart disease, and cancer than people who store excess fat around their hips and thighs.

Should you have an expanded waist line, it is critical that you follow the **Better Life Diet** guidelines given in this book.

We can learn much about the importance of diet and habits from studies of select population groups. For example:

Seventh-Day Adventists who restrict or avoid meat, tobacco, and alcohol have much less heart disease, emphysema, lung cancer, and liver disease than do people in the general population.

Deaths from breast and colon cancer are uncommon in countries where the diet is low in saturated (animal) fat.

Japanese emigrants to the U.S. who adopt the low-fiber carbohydrate, high-refined sugar, high-saturated fat, and high-*trans* fatty acid Western diet are at higher risk to develop coronary heart disease, diabetes, and breast and colon cancer than are the Japanese in Japan who eat their traditional high-fiber carbohydrate, low-refined sugar, low-saturated fat, and low-*trans* fatty acid native diet.

Compared with people of normal weight, obese people have a higher incidence of adult-onset diabetes, heart attacks, strokes, limb loss, cancer (prostate and breast), and gall bladder disease.

Comparable Servings for Different Food Groups

Fruits
- 1 whole medium sized fruit like an apple, pear, or peach (about 1 cup)
- 1/4 cup dried fruit
- 1/2 cup canned fruit
- 1/2 to 3/4 cup of unsweetened fruit juice

Vegetables & Legumes

- 1/2 cup cooked vegetables or legumes
- 1/2 cup raw chopped vegetables
- 1 cup raw leafy vegetables
- 1/2 to 3/4 cup vegetable juice

Pastas, Breads & Cereals (whole grain)

- 1/2 cup cooked pasta
- 1 slice bread
- 1 medium muffin
- 1/2 small bagel or English muffin
- 4 small crackers
- 1 small tortilla
- 1/2 cup cooked cereal
- 1/2 cup cooked rice

Milk & Milk Products

- 1 cup (8 oz.) low-fat milk or yogurt
- 1 slice low-fat cheddar cheese, 1/8" thick (1 oz.)
- 1 cup of low-fat cottage cheese

Meat & Meat Alternatives

- 2 to 3 oz. (size of a deck of cards) cooked *lean* meat, skinless poultry, or fish*
- 2 eggs **
- 7 oz. tofu
- 1 cup cooked legumes (dried beans or peas)
- 1/2 cup nuts or seeds
- Two tablespoons of natural peanut butter (no hydrogenation)

*   **The omega-3 oil in fish, especially salmon, tuna, and trout, is protective of your arteries. Next to flaxseed oil, fish oil contains the largest quantity of these valuable polyunsaturated fatty acids. Eat fish frequently (p. 67).**

**   **One to two eggs per day are good for you unless you are diabetic or have high blood values for LDL cholesterol and/or triglycerides. In that case we recommend that you limit eggs to 3-4/week. The liver makes about 3000 mg of cholesterol/day. One egg contains about 250 mg of cholesterol.**

How Many Servings Do **You** Need Each Day?

Calorie Level[1]	Children, Women, Older Adults About 1,600	Teen Girls, Active Women, Most Men About 2,200	Teen Boys, Active Men* About 2,800
Fruit Group	2	3	4
Vegetable and Legume Group	3	4	5
Bread, Cereal & Pasta Group	6	9	11
Milk & Milk Products Group[2]	2 to 4	3 to 5	4 to 6
Meat & Meat Alternatives Group	2	3	4
Total Fat (grams) [3]	53	73	93

* **Girls and women of comparable size, muscle mass, and activity level need the same number of calories as their male counterparts.**

1. **Servings of the major food groups** required at different calorie levels for the **Better Life Diet** (pp. 5,6).

2. **Teens, young adults, pregnant and nursing women, and women concerned about osteoporosis prevention** need the higher number of servings (or additional calcium from alternative sources).

3. **Number of grams of fat when 30% of daily calories are from fat sources.**

20 Ways to Lower
the Saturated Fat and *Trans* Fatty Acid
Content of Your Diet

1. Microwave, bake, broil (on rack), poach, braise, or stir-fry foods instead of frying whenever possible.

2. Use nonstick olive or canola cooking spray and a nonstick frying pan instead of adding butter or margarine.

3. Cook bacon and other fatty breakfast meats well, and then press them firmly between absorbent paper towels to remove as much of the remaining fat as possible.

4. Buy red meat with the least fat. "Prime" grade has the most fat, "choice" less, and "select" still less.

5. Purchase hamburger that is labeled "extra lean" and cook it well under the broiler to remove saturated fat.

6. Trim away all visible fat from meat before cooking and eating. This step can remove hundreds of calories.

7. Reduce the amount of saturated fat in canned meats, broths, and stews by chilling the cans before opening them. This causes the fat to rise to the top and solidify, making it easy to skim off.

8. Prepare foods in which the fat cooks into the liquid (stews, boiled meats, and soup stock) a day ahead of time. Then chill the food and remove the saturated fat which rises to the top and hardens.

9. Broil meats on a rack rather than frying them because the juices and liquified fat will collect in the pan below.

10. Defat these drippings if you make gravy with them by adding ice cubes to the drippings. This causes the fat to solidify and cling to the ice cubes.

11. Limit red meat to three 3-ounce servings (size of a deck of cards) of lean varieties a week. Eat more fish, poultry (without skin), eggs, legumes, nuts, seeds, and nonfat/low-fat dairy foods.

12. Remove the skin before cooking poultry because most of the fat is in, or just under, the skin.

13. Eat turkey year-round, not just at Thanksgiving. White meat eaten without the skin is best. It's low in fat.

14. Substitute mustard, ketchup, relish, mayonnaise, and/or salsa for butter and margarine in sandwiches.

15. Enjoy low-fat yogurt or nonfat sour cream on potatoes instead of butter or magarine.

16. Employ canola or olive oil for cooking and salads because they contain more protective monounsaturated and polyunsaturated fatty acids than other dietary fat (except flaxseed oil which cannot be used for cooking).

17. Switch from whole milk or reduced-fat milk to low-fat or nonfat milk. Whole milk will taste unbearably thick and fatty once you've become accustomed to nonfat milk. Your taste preference will change in several weeks.

18. Remember that an "imitation" product may have as much "bad" fat as the natural product if it is based on hydrogenated and/or tropical oils. Read the labels.

19. Choose the softer margarines because they have fewer *trans* fatty acids. Squeezable margarines have the least and stick margarines the most. Tub margarines have an intermediate amount of these "bad" fatty acids (pp. 66-68,71).

20. Select low-fat ("light," "diet," or "part-nonfat") cheeses, instead of regular whole milk cheeses.

Basics for Weight Control

The body can store little extra protein or carbohydrates, whereas it can store almost limitless quantities of fat in the cells of the adipose tissue. All carbohydrates are converted into glucose. Glucose stimulates the pancreas to secrete insulin which rapidly converts any excess glucose (that not needed for energy and unable to be stored as glycogen) into saturated fat. Less than a pound of glycogen can be stored in the entire body, 1/3 in the liver and 2/3 in the muscles. High insulin levels block the use of fat for energy. This creates a one way street -- fat in, no fat out.

But if low-fiber carbohydrates are markedly restricted and sugar is drastically reduced, weight reduction becomes relatively easy for most people - - if combined with a consistent, sensible exercise program (pp. 27-53). This dietary restriction reduces the insulin levels and enables the excess fat stores to be used for the energy needs of the body (p. 8). At the same time, exercise increases energy needs and speeds fat loss (see p. 51). The **Better Life Diet** and **Exercise Program** is also ideal for people with Syndrome X (see p. 71).

The **Better Life Diet** provides a balanced intake of carbohydrates, **50%** (mainly high-fiber varieties), fats, **30%** (mostly unsaturated types), and proteins, **20%** (those with little associated saturated fat) to supply the energy, building materials, fiber, minerals, phytochemicals, vitamins, and water needed by our bodies. If we need to gain weight, we eat more; if we need to lose weight, we eat less and exercise more; if we need to maintain weight, we continue as we are.

The building block diagram of the **Better Life Diet** on page 7 is a guide for developing such a balanced diet. The number of servings that you require of each of the main food groups depends on the extent of your caloric needs. (p. 11)

Achieving and Maintaining Your Ideal Weight

Each person has an "ideal" weight. We are all different. It makes no medical sense to try to "be like" someone else. We should all strive to achieve the body weight which is the most healthful for our particular physiological makeup. When you follow the **Better Life Diet** and **exercise program**, your body will self-regulate over a few weeks to many months to your ideal weight and then remain there so long as you stay with the program.

Too many Americans are obese. Obesity (excessive accumulation of saturated fat) makes the heart work harder, produces biochemical changes that cause arteries to harden and wear out, and predisposes us to adult-onset diabetes. Even losing only a few pounds of excess fat and keeping these pounds off is important.

Many people eat too much, don't exercise enough, and put on excess weight (fat). Losing this fat requires an action plan to **add muscle and lose excess fat** by eating the right foods in the proper amounts and by exercising every day.

Weight Loss Strategy
Crash diets *aren't* the answer. In the almost inevitable relapses that follow such diets, much more fat is added than muscle. The result is a fatter and weaker person who wonders what went wrong.

If you are overweight, there is a pleasant solution for your problem: start the **Better Life Diet** and at the same time work up over the next month to briskly walking two miles daily. If after a month you wish to lose weight at a faster rate, increase your walking program over the next month to four miles daily and don't eat *any* low-fiber carbohydrates or refined sugar while adhering to the rest of your dietary plan.

On this accelerated program you will lose 1/2 to 1 pound *more* per week. When you reach your target weight, continue the **Better Life Diet** (p. 5, and Fig. 2, p. 6) and **exercise program** at a level where you will look and feel your best, indefinitely.

Excess weight is saturated fat waiting to be used for energy. The two requirements to begin the fat burning process are:
  1. Consume fewer calories than you use.
  2. Decrease your insulin secretion by markedly restricting low-fiber carbohydrates and drastically reducing refined sugar in your diet. These reductions enable your fat stores to be used for energy (pp. 5,8,14).

When you combine these basic dietary requirements with a good exercise program, your body will automatically add muscles and shed those unwanted pounds of excess fat.

Weight Gain Strategy
Far more people need to lose rather than gain weight. Twenty % of Americans are seriously overweight. But being very thin is dangerous, too. Such people have essentially no glycogen, very little fat, and if they become ill and unable to eat, they must burn up their meager muscles for energy. If you need to gain weight, follow the **Better Life Diet**, and eat four to five meals a day instead of the customary three. Take a pleasant walk daily, increasing the distance as you gain needed weight. If you are even more severely underweight, please see your physician promptly.

A note about alcohol: If alcohol is consumed, it should be in moderation. In addition to the adverse effects of excess quantities on the brain and liver, alcohol is calorie rich (7 calories per gram) and is used by the body before glucose or fatty acids. Alcohol stops these normal metabolic processes. This makes weight control difficult.

Section II:
The Better Life Diet©
Sample Seven day Meal Plan and Nutritional Analysis
Anna Martin, and *Evette M. Hackman*, Ph.D., R.D., Department of
Consumer Science, Seattle Pacific University

Some comments about following The Better Life Diet menu:
• Eating well should progressively become a way of life for you. Your body and mind will respond positively to the changes you are making. Please note, however, that fiber intake should be increased gradually in order to avoid the unpleasant side effects of a sudden "fiber overload," for example: gas, bloating, and abdominal cramping.

• As you look at the nutrition information for each day, you can see that eating is not an exact science. There will be some variation in your daily food intake and calorie distribution. Your goal should be to meet The Better Life Diet 50/30/20 calorie percentages for carbohydrates, fats, and proteins by the week's end rather than on a daily basis. Also, this meal plan has been constructed for a 2000 calorie diet. Your needs may be smaller or greater (p. 11).

• Under the nutrition information, the total sugar count includes naturally occurring sugars (found in fruits, some vegetables, and milk, p.9) as well as added refined sugar. For each day of the menu, the refined sugar comprises no more than 10% of the total sugar count. Also, for each day of the menu, the combined saturated fatty acids (SFAs) and *trans* fatty acids (TFAs) comprise no more than 10% of the total calories.

• Nuts & Nut Butters: Nutritionally, the best choices of nuts are peanuts, almonds, and walnuts, but do not feel restricted to these choices. When shopping for natural nut butters, look at the ingredient list. Peanut butter, for example, should read peanuts and salt only. Other varieties of nut butters are available at natural food stores, including almond, cashew, hazelnut, macadamia, and more.

• **These menus were designed as guidelines to help you learn how to eat well and enjoy! Please view them as examples rather than the rule.** Here are some other marvelous resources to help you on your way:

1. *The Art of Nutritional Cooking, 2nd edition* by Michael Baskette and Eleanor Mainella. Upper Saddle River, NJ: Prentice-Hall, Inc.; 1999.

2. *Sunset Quick, Light, and Healthy* by the editors of Sunset Books. Menlo Park, CA: Sunset Publishing Corporation;1996.

3. *Cooking Light Magazine* by Doug Crichton, ed. Also, try visiting them on the web at www.cookinglight.com.

• Throughout the menu, when no beverage is specified you may choose to enjoy water, coffee, tea, diet soda, or any non-caloric drink.

B = breakfast   **L** = lunch   **Sn** = snack   **D** = dinner

DAY 1 (vegetarian)

B: French Toast
> 2 pieces wheat berry bread
> 2 whole eggs
> cinnamon to taste
> topped with:
>> 2 tsp butter
>> 1/2 cup fresh berries
> 1/2 cup fruit juice
> 8 oz nonfat light yogurt

L: Garden Burger
> 1 vegetable burger
> 1 whole grain hamburger bun topped with:
>> 1 tsp each: catsup, honey mustard, mayonnaise
>> 1/2 oz reduced fat cheese
>> 2-3 slices of tomato
>> 2-3 leaves of spinach
> 1 oz blue corn tortilla chips
> 1/4 cup salsa
> 1 cup nonfat milk

Sn: Fruit Smoothie
> 3 oz soft tofu
> 1/2 mango
> 1/2 banana, frozen
> 1/2 cup guava nectar
> 1 packet Equal® sweetener
> 2 Tbsp nuts of choice

> **The Better Life Diet meets the nutritional needs for the vast majority of Americans in a tasteful, satisfying, and healthy manner (pp. 5-8).**

D: Curried Lentil Soup
> 1 cup water with vegetable broth added
> 1/2 cup dry lentils
> 1/8 cup each: diced potato, carrot, celery, onion
> 1/8 tsp each: ginger, garlic, curry powder
> 1 1/2 tsp olive oil
> 1 medium slice wheat loaf bread oven-baked with
>> 1/2 oz reduced fat cheese, shredded
> 1 cup spiced coffee (add dash of cinnamon & nutmeg before brewing)
> 1 small almond biscotti, 3-inch size

Nutrition Information: Day 1
Total Cal: 2043, % Carbo: 53, % Fat: 28, % Pro: 19, SFA+TFA: 8.7%
> Total fiber: 46 g, Total sugars: 100 g (≤ 10% is refined)

DAY 2

B: Cold Cereal
> 1 cup Cheerios®
> 1/2 cup nonfat milk
> 1 banana, sliced
> 1/2 cup nonfat cottage cheese topped with
> 1 Tbsp each: raisins, sunflower seeds
> 1 cup fruit juice

L: Fish Soft Taco
> 2 oz halibut dipped in lime juice and bread crumbs, then broil
> cabbage slaw: 1/2 cup cabbage, 2 tsp mayonnaise, pepper & rice
> vinegar to taste
> 1 large garlic & herb flavored tortilla
> 2 Tbsp salsa
> fresh cilantro to taste
> 1/2 cup egg drop soup
> 8 oz nonfat light yogurt
> 2 persimmons

> **The Better Life Diet supplies all the daily requirements for minerals and vitamins.* (see pp. 25,26)**

Sn: Hummus with Pita
> 1/2 wheat pita pocket, cut into 4 wedges
> top each wedge with:
> > 2 Tbsp hummus
> > 1 each: tomato slice, cucumber slice, fresh mint leaf

D: Grilled Vegetable & Ham Sandwich
> 1 medium sized whole wheat hoagie roll
> 1 oz ham, deli meat
> 1 cup grilled vegetables: eggplant, squash, tomatoes, mushrooms,
> > bell peppers
> 1 oz Havarti cheese spread on roll:
> > 1 Tbsp plain nonfat yogurt
> > 1/2 tsp Dijon mustard
> > 1-2 cloves roasted garlic
> > 1 tsp olive oil
> 1/2 cup nonfat cottage cheese
> 1 cup watermelon slush, blend together:
> > 1 cup watermelon cubes, frozen
> > 1 packet Equal® sweetener
> > 1 1/2 Tbsp lemonade, frozen concentrate

Nutrition Information: Day 2
Total Cal: 1983, % Carbo: 53, % Fat: 26, % Pro: 22, SFA+TFA: 6%
> Total fiber: 36 g, Total sugars: 143 g ($\leq$ 10% is refined)

* For additional protection, we advise supplements (pp.28,61).

DAY 3

B: Vegetable Omelet
>   2 whole eggs
>   1 cup diced vegetables: tomatoes, bell peppers, mushrooms,
>   onions
>   1/2 oz reduced fat cheese
>   2 Tbsp salsa
>   2 pieces whole wheat toast topped with
>   2 oz herbed yogurt cheese*
>   1 orange

L: Quick & Easy Bagel
>   1 whole wheat bagel, halved & toasted, topped with:
>   2 Tbsp natural peanut butter
>   1 banana, sliced
>   1 cup nonfat milk

Sn: Trail Mix
>   1/2 cup Wheat Chex® cereal
>   1/4 cup assorted dry fruit
>   2 Tbsp nuts/seeds of choice
>   8 oz nonfat light yogurt

> **People who need less than 2,000 calories a day, especially women, should maintain a high milk, yogurt, and cheese intake to provide necessary calcium.**

D: Salmon
>   3 oz salmon fillet
>   marinate in 1/4 cup soy sauce, fresh ginger & garlic to
>   taste, then bake
>   1/2 cup steamed asparagus tips
>   topped with 1 tsp butter
>   1/2 yam, sliced and oven grilled
>   topped with 1 tsp butter
>   2/3 cup nonfat, sugar free ice cream topped with:
>   1/4 cup fresh berries
>   2 Tbsp chopped nuts of choice

Nutrition Information: Day 3
Total Cal: 2078, % Carbo: 53, % Fat: 27, % Pro: 20, SFA+TFA: 7%
      Total fiber: 45 g, Total sugars: 100 g (≤ 10% is refined)

*Note: Yogurt cheese can easily be made by straining plain yogurt overnight in the refrigerator through either a very fine mesh strainer or cheesecloth. Discard the liquid portion and season the cheese as desired (i.e.: sun-dried tomatoes, onion & dill, roasted garlic & thyme - - be imaginative).

DAY 4

B: Breakfast Sandwich
>   1 whole wheat English muffin, toasted
>   1 whole egg, fried with non-stick spray
>   2 pieces turkey bacon
>   1/2 oz reduced fat cheese
> 1 orange
> 1 cup nonfat milk

L: Quick Three Bean Chili
>   1 Lean Cuisine Three Bean Chili® entree
>   1/2 oz reduced fat cheese
>   2 tsp light sour cream
> 1 piece jalapeño corn bread, from mix
>   topped with 1 tsp butter
> 1 cup watermelon
> 1 cup nonfat milk

> **The Better Life Diet provides healthy food with great taste for a long life.**

Sn: Filled Tortilla
> 1/4 cup cooked black beans
> 1/8 cup cooked brown rice
> 1 oz reduced fat cheese
> 2 Tbsp salsa
> 1 whole wheat tortilla filled, folded, and fried in 1 tsp olive oil
> 2 tsp light sour cream

D: Pork Kabob
> marinade: 1/2 cup apple juice, 1 Tbsp olive oil, cloves, garlic, herbs
> marinate the following, then skewer with two bamboo spears & grill:
>   2 oz pork tenderloin, cubed
>   1/2 cup potato, cubed
>   1/2 cup asparagus tips
>   1/2 apple, cubed
>   4 pearl onions
> 1/2 cup cooked brown & wild rice
> 1 cup nonfat milk
> 1 Dole® fruit juice bar

Nutrition Information: Day 4
Total Cal: 2010, % Carbo: 50, % Fat: 28, % Pro: 22, SFA+TFA: 10%
      Total fiber: 35 g, Total sugars: 91 g (≤ 10% is refined)

DAY 5

B: Oatmeal
    1 cup cooked oatmeal stir in:
        2 Tbsp natural peanut butter
        1 packet Equal® sweetener
    1 apple
    1 cup nonfat milk

L: Turkey Sandwich
    2 pieces rye bread
    1 oz skinless turkey breast
    top with:
        1/2 oz reduced fat cheese
        1/4 of an avocado
        1 tsp Dijon mustard
        spinach, tomato, red onion, black olives
    2 kiwi
    1 cup nonfat milk

> **The Better Life Diet provides delicious food at low cost.**

Sn: English Muffin Pizza
    1 whole wheat English muffin, toasted
    top each half with:
        2 Tbsp spaghetti sauce
        1/2 vegetarian sausage link, sliced
        1/4 oz reduced fat cheese

D: Peanut Chicken Stir Fry
        3 oz skinless chicken breast
        1 cup stir fried vegetables (snap peas, bell pepper, zucchini,
            carrots, broccoli, mushrooms)
        1 cup brown rice
    peanut sauce - heat in saucepan then pour over stir fry dish:
        2 Tbsp each: Teriyaki sauce, natural peanut butter
        1/4 tsp each: ginger, crushed red pepper
        1 tsp sesame oil
    1 fortune cookie
    1 cup Lipton® spiced chai tea, made with equal parts nonfat milk &
        water
    1 packet Equal® sweetener

Nutrition Information: Day 5
Total Cal: 2038, % Carbo: 50, % Fat: 29, % Pro: 21, SFA+TFA: 6.1%
    Total fiber: 45 g, Total sugars: 88.6 g (≤ 10% is refined)

DAY 6

B: Breakfast Shake & Bagel
    1/2 banana, frozen
    1/2 cup each: frozen strawberries, orange juice, lowfat buttermilk
    1/2 tsp each: vanilla extract, nutmeg
  1/2 whole wheat bagel
  1 Tbsp almond butter

L: Pita Sandwich & Soup
    1/2 wheat pita pocket stuffed with:
      2 oz skinless chicken breast
      fresh spinach & artichoke hearts
      1 oz feta cheese
      red pepper pureé, blend together & spread inside pita:
        2 oz water packed roasted red pepper
        2 tsp olive oil
        1 tsp each: fresh parsley, capers, minced garlic
  1 Nile Spice® Instant Minestrone cup of soup
  1 orange
  1 cup nonfat milk

Sn: Tuna & Crackers
    1/4 cup tuna mixed with:
      2 Tbsp chopped celery
      2 tsp mayonnaise
  8 Triscuits®
  1 apple

> **Crash diets aren't the answer. The *Better Life Diet* with a good exercise program is the answer (pp. 14-16).**

D: Spaghetti With Meat Sauce
    1 cup vegetable sauce with:
      1/2 cup tomatoes
      1/4 cup each: zucchini, mushrooms
      Italian spices to taste
      1 tsp olive oil
  2 oz extra lean ground beef
  1 1/2 cup wheat spaghetti noodles
  top pasta dish with
    1 Tbsp each: pine nuts, parmesan cheese
  1/2 baked pear

Nutrition Information: Day 6
Total Cal: 2012, % Carbo: 53, % Fat: 28, % Pro: 19, SFA+TFA: 7.4%
    Total fiber: 42 g, Total sugars: 98 g (≤ 10 % is refined)

DAY 7 (fast food)

B: McDonald's
    1/2 Apple Bran Muffin
    1 serving pork sausage
    1 carton orange juice
    1 carton milk, 1 % *

L: Wendy's
    Grilled Chicken Sandwich
    Deluxe Garden Salad, nonfat dressing
    1 apple**
    1 carton milk, 2 % *

Sn: Muffin & Yogurt
    1/2 Apple Bran Muffin (from breakfast)
    8 oz nonfat light yogurt**
    1 small box raisins**
    1/2 cup baby carrots**

> **Combine the Better Life Diet with two miles of continuous brisk walking each day (pp. 40,41).**

D: Pizza Hut
    2 pieces Veggie Lover's pizza
    1 orange**

Nutrition Information: Day 7
Total Cal: 1894, % Carb: 51, % Fat: 30, % Pro: 19, SFA+TFA: 10%
    Total fiber: 20.3 g, Total sugars: 128 g (≤ 10% is refined)

* Nonfat milk would be best. The milk designated is the type that was sold at these fast food stores at the time of the writing of these meal guidelines.

** indicates items that must be brought from home

Note: This menu was included as an example of how to order a balanced meal on the rare occasion that you do eat out at a fast food restaurant. As you can see, you do not need to totally eliminate these foods from your diet. Fast foods, however, tend to be low in fiber and high in low-fiber carbohydrates, refined sugar, saturated fats, *trans* fatty acids, and sodium. In addition, your body does not get enough fresh fruits and vegetables when you eat out frequently.

7 Day Averages
of
Nutrients, Vitamins, and Minerals
for
Sauvage
Better Life Diet©

U.S. Label - - Adult

Basic Components

Calories	2008.56	
Calories from Fat	570.08	97%
Protein	106.55 g	213%
Carbohydrates	271.82 g	91%
Dietary Fiber	37.68 g	151%
Soluble Fiber	7.50 g	
Sugar - Total	107.84 g	
Monosaccharides	29.62 g	
Disaccharides	36.47 g	
Other Carbohydrates	102.46 g	
Fat - Total	63.34 g	97%
Saturated Fat	17.00 g	85%
Mono Fat	21.64 g	
Poly Fat	9.87 g	
Trans Fatty Acids	0.48 g	
Cholesterol	283.42 mg	94%
Water	1619.35 g	

Vitamins

Vitamin A (RE)	1587.21 (RE)	159%
A - Carotenoid	841.68 (RE)	
A - Retinol	340.02 (RE)	
A - Beta Carotene	4201.12 mcg	
Thiamin-B1	1.66 mg	111%

Riboflavin-B2	1.99 mg	117%
Niacin-B3	21.06 mg	105%
NiacinEquivalent	33.25 mg	166%
Vitamin-B6	2.07 mg	103%
Vitamin-B12	3.72 mcg	109%*
Vitamin C	211.73 mg	353%
Vitamin D	5.51 mcg	55%
Vitamin E-Alpha Equiv.	9.71 mg	108%
Folate	341.33 mcg	85%
Panothenic Acid	5.74 mg	57%

* Food Label Value

Minerals

Calcium	1451.68 mg	145%
Copper	1.52 mg	76%
Iron	16.94 mg	94%
Magnesium	366.93 mg	92%
Manganese	4.74 mg	
Phosphorus	1478.80 mg	148%
Potassium	3831.87 mg	109%
Selenium	99.21 mcg	
Sodium	2608.52 mg	109%
Zinc	9.40 mg	63%

Other Fats

Omega-6 Fatty Acids	7.03 g
Omega-3 Fatty Acids	0.69 g

Ratio - 10:1 **

Other

Alcohol	0.21 g
Caffeine	19.64 ng

** A ratio of 4:1 or a little less is better. Taking one teaspoon daily of pleasant tasting flaxseed oil (richest source of omega-3 fatty acids) would reduce the ratio to 2.5:1. I take one teaspoon daily of Barleans Lignan Rich Flax Oil from Barleans Organic Oils, 4936 Lake Terrell Road, Ferndale, WA 98248. Phone 800-445-3529.

Section III:
Exercise - - Essential Ally of Diet

To benefit your body, exercise must be **aerobic** ("with oxygen"). If you can carry on a normal conversation while exercising, that exercise is aerobic for you. Aerobic exercise *doesn't* deplete your muscles of oxygen, make you short of breath and unable to talk, or cause you to perspire heavily (unless it's very warm). On the other hand, **anaerobic** ("without oxygen") exercise *does* deplete your muscles of oxygen, make you breathless and unable to speak, and cause you to perspire heavily.

Anaerobic exercise demands more oxygen and nutrients than the arterial blood can deliver to the overworked muscles. It also produces more waste products than the blood can remove. This excessive exercise makes you severely short of breath, causes your pulse to race, and wears you out quickly. It's neither good nor safe for the average person.

Aerobic exercise, however, is rhythmic muscular activity performed at a pace within the capacity of the circulation to deliver the extra oxygen and nutrients the working muscles need. The blood also removes carbon dioxide and other waste products. You can continue this exercise for long periods with a stable, moderately elevated pulse rate without becoming breathless, exhausted, or drenched in sweat. Aerobic exercise is safe and good for you. It's the exercise you need to become healthy and stay that way.

The ability to talk while exercising (the talk test) is a simple way to tell whether an exercise is "aerobic" for you. If you can carry on a normal conversation, it is; if you can't, it's anaerobic. People in poor shape fail the test while walking

27

slowly; people in good shape pass while walking briskly; people in excellent shape pass while jogging. Regardless of the activity, adjust your pace so you can pass the "test."

Aerobic exercise:

- Costs little in time or money.
- Increases your enjoyment of life.
- Tones your muscles.
- Sharpens your mind.
- Reduces stress.
- Alleviates depression.
- Promotes sound sleep.
- Strengthens your heart and lungs.
- Assists your whole body to use oxygen and nutrients more efficiently.
- Helps your digestive system work better,
- Improves dangerous blood chemistry.

Regular aerobic exercise also acts to help women after menopause prevent or at least slow down the development of osteoporosis, a process that absorbs bone structure and weakens the skeleton. The protective effect of exercise is enhanced by the *Better Life Diet* and by taking Vitamin D, calcium, magnesium, and estrogen.

Severe osteoporosis weakens the long bones so much that they break easily, especially the hip, and makes the backbone so fragile that portions of it may collapse. Even without obvious fractures, osteoporosis silently shortens the spine with age and causes both men and women to lose height as they get older.

We all need aerobic exercise to help lose excess fat, strengthen muscles, improve heart and lung function, gain a renewed sense of vigor; and avoid developing adult-onset diabetes, blindness, kidney failure, high blood pressure, hardening of the arteries, heart attacks, strokes, decreased walking capacity, limb loss, aneurysms, and hemorrhages.

In brief, regular aerobic exercise is the closest thing we have to an "anti-aging pill." You'll find that life's a lot more fun when you take this "pill" every day.

Walking briskly without becoming winded is hard to beat as an exercise for many reasons. It's safe, pleasant, inexpensive, good for most everything, and able to be enjoyed nearly any time and any place. Try it! Two miles in the morning or evening will do wonders for you. This is a habit to form and practice for life.

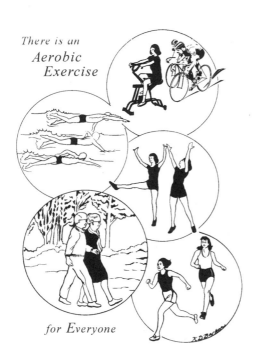

There is an *Aerobic Exercise* ... *for Everyone*

Walk with your husband, wife, children, friend, or dog. If none of them are available, walk alone. This is time you owe yourself. Precious time.

If you can't walk two miles, try one. If not one, do what is comfortable for you and slowly increase the distance.

Figure 3 -- Aerobic exercise ("with oxygen") is good "every day medicine." But if you are seriously overweight or have heart trouble or other illness, please contact your physician for guidance before beginning an exercise program.

F.I.T.

The Basics - Think F.I.T.

The first thing to know about "regular aerobic exercise" is that unless you do it *frequently enough, intensely enough,* and *long enough,* it's not going to do you, your cardiovascular and respiratory systems, or your weight reduction program much good.

As an aid to getting in shape and staying that way, think F.I.T. for the **frequency**, **intensity**, and **time** of exercise.

Frequency

The American College of Sports Medicine recommends daily aerobic exercise. We need to use our muscles consistently to keep them and our heart and lungs in shape. There's no way around this requirement. We either use our muscles or we lose them -- an easy choice if we wish to get in shape and stay that way.

Intensity

Most of the mystique that surrounds aerobic exercise has to do with its intensity, or "pace."

Take the "talk test" to find the aerobic pace that's right for you (p. 27,28). Increase your pace to where you can't carry a conversation and then slow down to where you can. In doing this, don't try to exercise on the "edge." Give yourself some "breathing room."

When you're in the "groove," you'll work up a moderate

sweat, but you won't get breathless. If you find yourself huffing and puffing and unable to carry on a conversation, slow down and find the pace that's right for you. Leave long distant running and triathlon competition to the athletes. It's not healthy for you to go to the edge of your endurance. Brisk walking is hard to beat. Try it! You'll be pleased. It works, and it's entirely safe.

Time

Studies show that for reasonable fitness, we need at least 30 minutes of aerobic exercise every day of the week.

There is some controversy here. A panel of experts convened by the American College of Sports Medicine and the Centers for Disease Control (CDC) recently announced that *accumulating* 30 minutes of "moderate exercise" each day (e.g., walking, gardening, climbing several flights of stairs and/or doing housework *every* day) is enough to improve overall fitness, at least moderately. Researchers at the Harvard School of Public Health, however, believe that 45 minutes of daily, brisk, *continuous* exercise is preferable.

The bottom line is that even a *little* exercise is better than no exercise, and in general, *more* exercise is better than less exercise -- within reason of course.

Thirty minutes of daily aerobic exercise will help you attain and maintain your optimal weight. If you need to lose weight faster, get 45 to 60 minutes of continuous aerobic exercise once, or, if necessary, twice a day. This need not be complicated. Just go out and start walking. You can build from there.

Questions and Answers
About Exercise

Q. *What are the different types of exercise?*

A. 1. Isometric exercise (muscle contraction without motion) tones your muscles, but doesn't move your body around. This type of exercise uses few calories and doesn't improve overall cardiovascular and muscular fitness.

2. Isotonic exercise -- such as weight lifting -- builds muscle tissue and uses calories but doesn't do enough to promote cardiovascular or pulmonary fitness.

3. Anaerobic exercise *(without* adequate oxygen) -- such as sprinting or fast cycling -- leads to exhaustion and breathlessness in a few minutes. This type of exercise can't be continued long enough for needed benefits to be realized. Also, anaerobic exercise can be dangerous because it quickly depletes your heart of oxygen.

4. Aerobic exercise *(with* adequate oxygen . . . if your pace is right) such as walking, dancing, jogging, golfing (preferably without a cart), cycling, swimming, handball, tennis, rowing, and rope skipping are the most popular. At a proper aerobic pace, these exercises build muscle, get your heart and lungs in shape, help you attain and maintain a healthful weight, and keep you in good condition. This combination of benefits could save your life.

Q. *Should I check with my doctor before beginning an exercise program?*

A. Yes, if you:
- Haven't seen your doctor for a long time.
- Are over 35 years of age.
- Have a personal or family history of cardiovascular disease.
- Are a smoker.
- Have high blood pressure.
- Are seriously overweight.

Q. *How do I know which aerobic exercise is best for me?*

A. Considerations for choosing an aerobic exercise (or a combination of aerobic exercises) should include:
- The availability or price of equipment purchase or rental.
- Your personal health, weight, and age.
- Your level of fitness.
- Your interests.
- The weather.
- How much time you have.

Special Note: It is important to find exercises that you *like* to do. Then you will feel good about sticking to your new exercise routine.

Q. *How can I find time to exercise?*

A. The same way you find time every day to eat and sleep. Exercise is just as important. Make it a priority.

Q. *What are my exercise choices?*

A. There are many. The following comments about the more popular aerobic exercises are to pique your interest and get you involved.

1. Aerobics

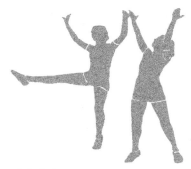

Special Advantages:

- Special fun for those who like exercising to music.
- Entire body is exercised.
- Group spirit is established in the classes.
- Necessary skill is rapidly acquired. Beginners become "pros" in a short time.
- Classes are held inside, away from the weather.
- Many styles of aerobics and different kinds of music to choose from.

Special Equipment/Facilities Needed:
- Loose-fitting clothing and comfortable shoes with cushioned soles (athletic shoes give the best support).
- Space and a qualified instructor.

Advice for Beginners:
- The best way to find a good aerobics program and instructor is by word-of-mouth referral. Talk to your friends and find out what program and which instructor they enjoy and why. If that doesn't work, check with the registered programs in your community such as those at the YWCA or YMCA and ask what they offer. Then talk to their instructors.

- Sign up for classes with a friend. You'll push each other and have a lot of fun doing so.

- The typical aerobic dance program consists of a one-hour class Monday, Wednesday, and Friday for three months. There are, however, aerobics classes that are only offered twice a week. These don't provide enough exercise to get your cardiovascular and respiratory systems in good shape. To get more exercise, sign up for two programs, or supplement your classes with other aerobic exercises that you do on your own, such as walking or swimming.

- Make sure you exercise strenuously enough in your class to work up a moderate sweat, but don't get so carried away that your pace causes you to become breathless and drenched in sweat.

2. Cycling

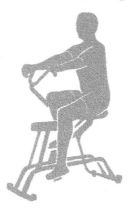

Special Advantages:
- Especially well-suited for older and overweight individuals, and for those with back, knee, and/or foot problems.

- Outdoor bikes can be used for transportation.

- Indoor bikes provide protection from the weather, and you can read or watch TV while exercising.

Special Equipment Needed:
- An outdoor or indoor bike. These may be purchased or rented from a cycle shop. Want ads and garage sales may be useful in finding a good second-hand bike.

- Before purchasing a bike, check consumer magazines, read a bicycle book, and talk with friends. If you still need more guidance, consult a fitness professional. Then comparison shop.

- Outdoor bikes should have at least three gears.

- Indoor bikes must have a tension control -- all other special features are optional.

Advice for Beginners:
- Work on finding a pedaling pace and tension control that will give you an adequate workout without causing shortness of breath. If you get to a point of breathlessness, slow down until you catch your breath. Then pick your pace up to the point you're sweating some but aren't winded.

- Have a bike specialist "fit" your bike to your body by adjusting the seat and handle bar heights and positions so your legs and back are comfortable.

- Outdoor cyclists should wear helmets because they provide needed protection which could prevent a devastating head injury in case of an accident.

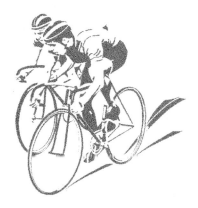

3. Swimming

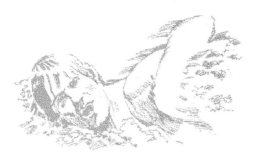

Special Advantages:
- Well-suited for everyone and especially those with back and/or joint problems which restrict or prohibit them from enjoying other popular aerobic exercises.

- The perfect aerobic exercise for those who want a good workout but hate to sweat.

- Works on all body muscles.

Special Equipment/Facilities Needed:
- Swim suit.

- Eye and ear protection, if necessary.

- A swimming pool. Check out the parks department pools, or the pool at the YMCA, YWCA, or local health club. Be sure that the pool you select is large enough for nonstop lap swimming.

Advice for Beginners:
- Inquire when your local pool opens for lane swimming. Some pools are open from 5:00 A.M. to 10:00 P.M.

- Use any stroke and get in as much nonstop lane swimming as possible during your exercise time. If you start to lose your breath, switch to a lazy sidestroke. Once you've caught your breath, find your proper stroke and pace.

- If it's difficult for you to get to a pool on a regular basis, use the other suggested aerobic exercises to supplement your swimming program.

Swimming and Osteoporosis:
- Studies have shown that swimming *doesn't* help strengthen bones. If you're concerned about osteoporosis, get plenty of *weight-bearing* exercise, like walking.

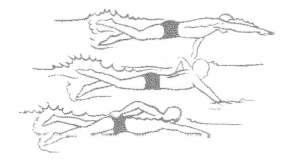

4. Walking

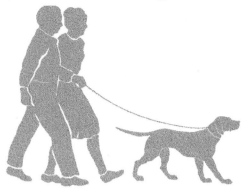

Special Advantages:
- Good way to begin an exercise program if you haven't been exercising, have special medical problems, and/or are overweight.

- Can be used to limber up sore muscles if you've "overdone it" with one of the other aerobic exercises.

- Can be used for transportation.

- Can provide the same benefits as jogging, with less risk of injury.

- No expertise needed; you've been doing it since you were one year old.

Special Equipment Needed:
- Comfortable shoes with cushioned soles.

Advice For Beginners:

- If you're out of shape, begin slowly and first increase the distance and then your pace, but do this in a careful, progressive manner. If you become breathless, you're going too fast . . . slow down! When you've caught your breath, continue at a pace that enables you to talk normally.

- Over a period of weeks to months, work up to a level where you can briskly walk nonstop for 30 to 60 minutes without feeling winded.

- Don't count the stop-and-go casual walking you do around the house or at the office as part of your walking program. Stop-and-go exercises don't provide significant conditioning benefits for your heart and lungs. Set aside special time for brisk, nonstop walking.

- Overweight people find that the addition of nonstop, brisk walking to their daily routines can help them lose weight without having to severely reduce their caloric intake.

- When you reach a point where you need more of a challenge, strap on a weighted backpack or add a few hills to your walking program.

- Notes on brisk-walking form: Swing your arms, take long strides, and look at the beautiful world around you.

5. Jogging

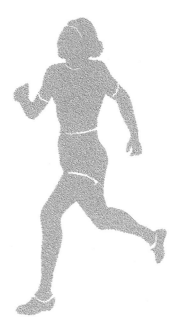

Special Advantages:

- The growing number of jogging trails and indoor/outdoor tracks make for great access and convenience. Concrete is not the best choice for a running surface (too hard), nor is grass (too bumpy).

- It's fun and motivating to jog with a companion if you like company during exercise. Pick a buddy, however, who's approximately at your level of fitness. If he or she is in much better shape, you will be run ragged. If your companion lags far behind in speed and/or stamina, you won't be able to get to the level of exercise that you need.

Special Equipment Needed:

- Quality running shoes (not sneakers) are a must to protect your feet and joints from the pounding they take in jogging. Shoes should extend 3/4" beyond the longest toe, fit perfectly over athletic socks, allow no slippage of the heel, be sufficiently flexible (even when new) to be comfortable, and have shock-absorbing soles.

- Hundreds of brands and varieties of running shoes are available. Shop around until you find a perfect fit. (Athletic stores tend to have wider selections and salespeople with more expertise.)

- Dress in layers when it's cold; don't overdress when it's warm.

- If you have knee and/or foot problems, you may need to see an orthopedist or a podiatrist to obtain special instructions and/or an orthotic shoe insert.

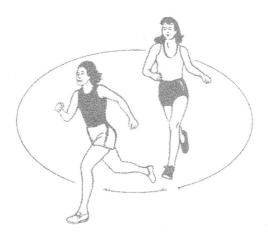

Beginning Jogging

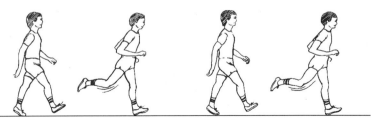

Alternate walking with slow jogging.

Advice for Beginners:

- At first, alternate walking with slow jogging, slowing to a walk whenever you reach the point where you can't talk normally. Gradually increase the proportion of jogging time to walking time until you are jogging on a nonstop basis. Don't expect too much too soon.

- If you feel you are able to do more, extend your time, not your speed (pace).

- Beginners should invest in a good book on jogging before beginning their program.

- Don't try to keep up with others who are in better shape than you. Exercise at your own pace.

- Take time to "warm up" and stay within your limits.
- Don't lean forward when you jog.
- Hold your forearms approximately parallel to the ground, and keep your hands and shoulders relaxed.
- Keep your strides short -- don't get your feet out ahead of your knees.
- Land on your heels, not on the balls of your feet.
- Breathe through your mouth.
- When you're within about 10 minutes of stopping jogging, begin to slow down gradually and finish by walking at a comfortable pace for several more minutes. This allows time for your circulation to clear the lactic acid from your muscles in order to avoid having them become stiff and sore.

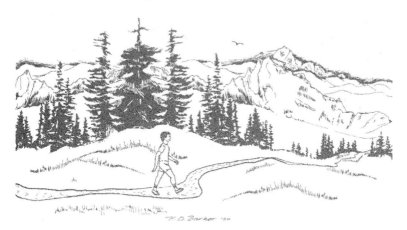

Times to Exercise

Before Breakfast

Advantages:

- Clears your mind and invigorates your body so you can begin your day with enthusiasm.
- At this refreshing time of day it's hard to make excuses for not exercising.
- You have to take a shower anyway.

Possible Disadvantages:

- It may be hard to get out of bed a little earlier.

Before Lunch

Advantages:

- Works off morning tensions.
- Refreshes you to meet the afternoon demands.
- Helps curb lunch appetite.

Possible Disadvantages:

- You've got to have a place to shower . . . or a lot of cologne.
- Your lunch break may not be long enough for you to get in an adequate exercise session and still have time for lunch, too.

Before Dinner

Advantages:

- Clears the day's tensions.
- Refreshes you for evening activities.
- Helps curb dinner appetite.

Possible Disadvantages:

- Easy to find a reason not to exercise at this time of day.

Before Bed

Advantages:

- Clears your mind and helps you relax.

Possible Disadvantages:

- Easy to say -- "It's late, I'll do it tomorrow."
- Need to wait until you feel up to exercising after you've finished eating.

There are a million excuses for not exercising regularly. Here are a few:

"I don't have the time."

All it takes is a minimum of 30 minutes of aerobic exercise daily to stay in reasonable shape. "Steal" 10 minutes from your usual TV watching time, 10 minutes from your sleep time, and 10 minutes from your goof-off time, and you'll be set.

"I don't have the energy."

The vast majority of people who exercise regularly say exercise makes them "feel full of energy," and that's why they do it. Exercise, by getting the blood circulating and the muscles moving, is an ideal way to overcome frustration, relieve stress, and clear your mind of the day's problems. In this way, it serves to supply you with more energy, providing a kind of "second wind."

"I always get sore."

Sore muscles come from doing too much, too soon, and not coming to a gradual stop. Start a routine where you gradually increase the time of exercising before increasing the speed (pace). And, before stopping, slow down gradually over 5 to 10 minutes, so your muscles won't become stiff and sore.

"It's too much work to get in shape."

A nice thing about aerobic exercise is that you can adjust the pace to suit your needs. You'll soon find the right speed that will allow you to progressively extend your exercise time to 30 minutes without becoming breathless.

"I've tried getting more exercise, but I never stick with it."

This time you will! You can afford 30 minutes of exercise every day of the week. No big deal. (If you need a motivator, exercise with a buddy, use gold stars on a calendar, or anything that works for you.) The key is to *make exercise a priority* and develop it into a faithful habit.

"I'm too old."

You're as old as you feel, and regular exercise makes you feel younger. Take it slowly, and work on *gradually* increasing your muscular, cardiovascular, and respiratory endurances.

"I hate fighting the weather."

An indoor swimming pool, exercycle, shopping mall (for walking), and an aerobics class can help. If these don't suit your fancy, get a treadmill and walk *inside* on rainy days.

"I have arthritis."

Your doctor will probably recommend that you swim or cycle indoors. Studies show that these exercises help relieve arthritic pains and stiffness.

"I'm too busy running around doing things for other people."

In order to help others more effectively, you must first take care of yourself. A half-hour of aerobic exercise every day is a gift you *must* give yourself. It will allow you to feel and look your best, while you do more for others.

"Exercise is boring!"

Well, see what you can do to make it "fun!" Vary your walking/jogging route. Listen to music. Position your indoor bike so you can watch the evening news while you pump away. Join an aerobic dance class. Exercise with a friend. Treat yourself to new athletic shoes. Challenge yourself.

"I don't know what to do with the kids."

If possible, take them with you (they need exercise, too!). There are walking/jogging strollers on the market for exercising with very young children. You can also invest in an indoor bike or treadmill. Many health clubs have child day-care facilities; check them out.

"My family isn't interested."

That's okay. This is something you're doing for yourself.

"I'm not that interested in fitness; I've got other priorities."

Stop for a moment and reflect, "Exercise will help me live longer and better." And that's for real! And there's more.

Difficult problems often "solve themselves" while you exercise. This isn't a trick. Exercise refreshes your mind and helps you think more clearly.

"I don't have the right clothes, equipment, etc."

Buy them. It could be one of the most valuable investments of your life.

"I'm too fat."

So . . . you're just the one who needs to exercise. Start with something easy, like walking around the block. Do that for a week. Go around twice the next week, and so on. See how much better you'll feel -- and how much less you'll want to eat! Keep at it, and you'll begin to feel better and better as you progressively lose excess fat while you gain needed muscle.

Exercise charts only tell half the story. First of all, many people find that regular aerobic exercise helps them curb their appetite. One reason for this is that exercise tends to reduce tension and depression, common causes of the "munchies." Exercise also signals the liver to convert some of its glycogen into glucose and release it into the blood, which helps curbs the appetite.

Second, muscles which are exercised on a regular basis use more energy (calories) even when resting than muscles which have not been exercised. Exercise "tunes" the body's engines (muscles) so they idle faster at rest.

In addition, fit people, pound per pound, burn more calories than fat people because a pound of resting muscle burns more calories than a pound of fat. This difference in caloric consumption becomes even more pronounced after exercising and lasts for many hours.

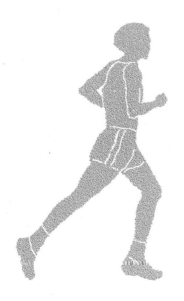

Have faith. If you have a large amount of fat to lose and are only losing 1/2-to-1 lb. per week, don't get discouraged. You're on track. Fifty pounds in a year is a lot. Remember, the right way to lose weight permanently is to lose excess fat gradually while you add muscle (pp. 14-16).

"I will just exercise the fat parts of my body"

It's true that fat tends to concentrate in specific areas of the body. It generally shows up on the hips and thighs of women, and around the waists of men.

Spot-reduction exercises like sit-ups and leg-lifts make those muscles stronger and firmer. The same fat deposits, however, still sit on top of these muscles. The fat on top of a muscle does not belong to that muscle; it belongs to the whole body. This fat will begin to "melt away" only when the demand for calories in the whole body exceeds the caloric intake.

Spot-reduction exercises don't demand a great deal of energy. Whole body aerobic exercises are better because they use large sets of muscles and require more calories to meet the increased energy requirements. And when you use more calories than you eat, you lose weight. Simple as that.

Special Note: It's not a particularly fond subject of mine, but there is a drastic solution some people try -- major plastic surgery to remove fat deposits. One such operation is called **liposuction**. The surgeon inserts a tubular suction device through the skin and uses it to slim and contour the excessively padded areas by literally sucking out the fat. Though this procedure is indicated for some patients, it's an **expensive and potentially dangerous way to lose fat**. If you are considering this method, I strongly encourage you to become well informed about all aspects of this surgery before you undergo this harsh treatment. There is a **better way** -- **The Better Life Diet** and **Exercise Program**!

"I had coronary bypass surgery three weeks ago, and I don't know if it's safe for me to begin an exercise program"

If you are gaining strength, feeling better, and able to walk up a flight or two of stairs without becoming short of breath or developing chest pain, your doctor will be delighted! He or she will likely start you on a progressive walking program following the guidelines given on pages 40 and 41.

In brief, your physician will monitor your progress and first extend the distance you walk and then increase the speed cautiously. He or she may also refer you to a cardiac rehabilitation program near your home. There are many good programs available today.

Exercise is an important part of both your short-term and long-term treatment plan. Don't become impatient and go too fast early on, or become too busy to exercise later on.

Remember, the time you take to exercise is a precious gift you owe yourself and your loved ones. Make your exercise program a high priority because it's so important to your having a long and youthful life from this point forward.

Section IV:

Simple Plan for a Long and Youthful Life

General Considerations 55-56

The Five Cardinal Rules for
Healthy Living 56-59

Three Additional Strategies 60-63

    1. Take Antioxidant and
       Homocysteine-Lowering Vitamins 61

    2. Reduce the Stickiness of
       Your Platelets if They Are
       Too Sticky 62

    3. Select a Good Doctor and
       Follow His or Her Advice 63

General Considerations

Heart attack and stroke are the leading killers in the industrial world. But the good news is that the death rate for cardiovascular disease in the U.S. has decreased about 20% in recent years even though the incidence of obesity and adult-onset diabetes has risen. There is much yet to do.

Hardening of the arteries (atherosclerosis) begins early in life. *Autopsy examinations of adolescent American accident victims show that most already have fatty plaques in their coronary arteries.* These findings indicate that we must start in childhood to prevent heart disease from developing. This can be done by teaching today's children the rules of healthy living in three interrelated ways:

1. Good example and instruction by parents in the home. This is vital!
2. Positive guidance by pediatricians and family physicians.
3. Proper training by teachers in the schools.

"An ounce of *prevention* in early years is worth a pound of *cure* in later years." But prevention efforts must be both *simple* and *effective* if they are to be widely adopted.

Our guidelines pass this test. They are: Don't smoke. Follow the **Better Life Diet**. Perform aerobic exercise every day. Attain and maintain a healthful weight. Control stress.

These guidelines will help you avoid developing hardening of the arteries, clots, heart attacks, strokes, decreased walking capacity, limb loss, high blood pressure, aneurysms, hemorrhages, many types of cancer (especially of the lung), emphysema, adult-onset diabetes, blindness, and kidney failure.

In addition, these guidelines are vital if you have had surgery for heart or artery disease. This is because surgery is only a *mechanical* solution to a structural problem. You also need to prevent the development of more atherosclerosis (p. 64).

Given enough time, all arteries will eventually wear out. In earlier years so many people died of infections (such as smallpox, pneumonia, influenza, typhoid, diphtheria, tuberculosis, staph infections, strep infections, meningitis, and appendicitis) that few lived long enough for this to happen. In fact, most people died before reaching age 50.

Now that we are living longer (the average life span in the U.S. is about 72 years for men and 78 for women), nearly *half* of us will die from hardened arteries and clots unless we take steps now to prevent this from happening later.

The Five Cardinal Rules
for
Healthy Living

To increase our chances of living to a ripe old age with our mental faculties and physical capabilities in top form, it's necessary to follow an effective plan to keep our arteries in good condition. Our plan may be expressed through the letters: **S ... D-E-W ... S** which identify the core subjects of the five cardinal rules for healthy living:

Smoking . . . **D**iet-**E**xercise-**W**eight . . . **S**tress.

A prime objective is to prevent the development of atherosclerosis which causes clots to form that block the flow channels of vital arteries. The program works in two main ways. *First,* it lowers the blood levels of LDL cholesterol, triglycerides, and homocysteine while elevating HDL cholesterol levels. *Second,* it decreases the blood's ability to clot by lowering the level of fibrinogen and by keeping platelets from becoming too sticky. This keeps vital blood flowing throughout our bodies. The cardinal rules are:

S*moking* • **Don't smoke**, or be around those who are smoking. This helps to prevent heart attacks, strokes, limb loss, cancer, and emphysema.

D*iet* • **Eat** a delicious diet consisting of high-fiber carbohydrates, protective fats, and good proteins. Severely restrict your intake of low-fiber carbohydrates, refined sugar, saturated fat, and *trans* fatty acids. This helps to prevent heart attacks, strokes, limb loss, hypertension, cancer, adult-onset diabetes, blindness, and kidney failure.

The **Better Life Diet** (pp. 1-26) reflects the general admonition that if a food grows in the ground or on trees, swims, or has feathers, it's good for you with a few exceptions.

E*xercise* • **Perform** at least 30 minutes of **daily aerobic exercise** (pp. 27-53).

W*eight* • **Attain and maintain** your **ideal weight**. This is the weight at which you feel and look your best.

S*tress* • **Strive** for the **inner peace** that allows you to willingly accept problems as a challenging part of normal life. You can best achieve this mental state free of harmful stress by freely helping those who need you in a spirit of unconditional love.

Rules for Healthy Living

S . . . D-E-W . . . S

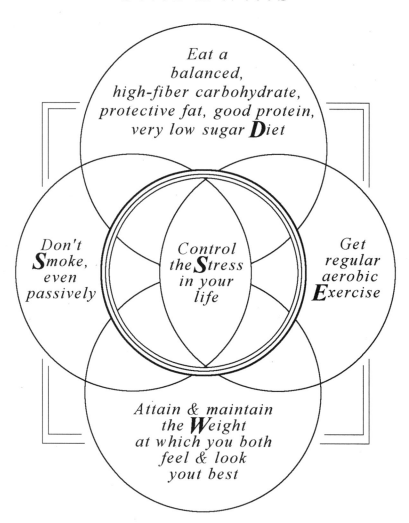

Eat a
balanced,
high-fiber carbohydrate,
protective fat, good protein,
very low sugar **D**iet

Don't
Smoke,
even
passively

Control
the**S**tress
in your
life

Get
regular
aerobic
Exercise

Attain & maintain
the **W**eight
at which you both
feel & look
yout best

*Figure 4 - The five interlocking rules for healthy living are vital
for a long and youthful life (for diet, see p. 5 & Fig. 2, p.6).*

Eat for Health and Taste
Protect Your Arteries
& Enjoy Life

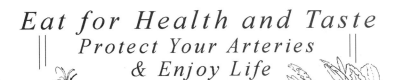

*Fresh fruits,
fresh vegetables,
& legumes*

*Fish &
poultry without skin*

Eggs,* may have 1-2 per day

Drink nonfat milk

*Whole grain breads, cereals,
& pastas*

---

*Markedly restrict low-fiber carbohydrates
(white bread, mashed potatoes,
french fries, & white rice)*

Drastically restrict refined sugar

*Severely restrict saturated fat,
and <u>trans</u> fatty acids*

** For people who don't have diabetes, cholesterol,
or triglyceride problems.
(For those who do, please see pp. 10 and 64-69)*

*Figure 5 - **The Better Life Diet** --
Delicious foods that are good for you.*

Three Additional Strategies

If people would follow the five cardinal rules for healthy living, the incidence of obesity, diabetes, blindness, kidney failure, cancer, hypertension, heart attacks, strokes, and limb loss would decrease dramatically. But some need more. These are the people who have a family or personal history of heart or artery disease at a young age (35-40 years) or have one or more of the following threatening blood chemistries:

1. An HDL cholesterol level below 30 mg/dL in men and below 40 mg/dL in women. The higher this value the better - - HDL transports LDL cholesterol out of the blood and the arterial wall.

2. A fasting blood glucose value above 120 mg/dL.

3. A fasting triglyceride level above 200 mg/dL. (Triglycerides are fats derived both from the fatty foods in our diet, and from the conversion of excess carbohydrates and proteins into saturated fat.)

4. An LDL cholesterol level above 150 mg/dL. The *ideal* value for this lipid is under 100 mg/dL.

5. A fibrinogen level above 350 mg/dL. (Fibrinogen forms clots -- a value of 200-250 mg/dL is ideal.)

6. A fasting platelet aggregation score above 30. (Sticky platelets cause blood to clot.)

7. Elevated levels of homocysteine. (see next page).

These people need the following three *additional strategies:*

1. Take Antioxidant and
Homocysteine-Lowering Vitamins

"Free radical" is a popular term used to explain nearly everything that goes wrong in the body from cancer to heart disease and from arthritis to cataracts. This term refers to oxygen atoms which have lost electrons. These electron-deficient (oxidized) atoms severely damage neighboring atoms by robbing them of their electrons.

Current theory suggests that only oxidized low-density lipoprotein cholesterol (LDL) damages the arterial wall. If proven true, the blood level of oxidized LDL will be important information to help predict an individual's risk of developing a heart attack.

Chemicals that prevent free radicals from doing damage are called "antioxidants." Of the foods with such properties (fruits, vegetables, legumes, nuts and seeds), blueberries have the most. In addition to enjoying a healthy, nutritious diet, protect yourself further against these "radicals" by taking 50 mg of Vitamin B6, 500 mg of Vitamin C, and 400 units of Vitamin E daily. And these vitamins only cost about 12 cents a day. Further, we suggest that people with multiple risk factors also take 30 mg of coenzyme Q-10 daily. This powerful antioxidant costs about 50 cents a day.

We also suggest that you take a multivitamin that has 0.4 mg of folic acid and 10 mcg of Vitamin B12. These vitamins along with Vitamin B6 reduce the blood level of *homocysteine,* an amino acid, which in high concentration (above 12 micromols/L) injures endothelial cells and predisposes the inner arterial wall to develop atherosclerosis. Smoking, inactivity, and other factors that cause atherosclerosis also increase homocysteine.

2. *Reduce the Stickiness of Your Platelets If They Are Too Sticky*

The degree of stickiness that platelets can develop is unique to each person. Platelets that become *very sticky* can cause fatal blood clots. Such platelets may *adhere, activate,* and *aggregate* on the diseased flow surface of atherosclerotic arteries, especially when soft plaques rupture and release their deadly lipid contents into the blood. These platelet aggregates may cause clots to form which can block the channel and stop the flow of blood to vital regions. Such lack of blood supply causes heart attacks, strokes, high blood pressure, blindness, kidney failure, decreased walking capacity, and gangrene of the feet and lower legs.

Life depends on an almost endless series of checks and balances of which the stickiness of our platelets is but one example. If our platelets couldn't stick together, we would *bleed to death.* But if they are too sticky, we would *clot to death.* What we want is the right balance.

Millions of people take an aspirin a day to reduce the stickiness of their platelets even though they don't know whether this is either necessary or effective for them. Studies at **The Hope Heart Institute** in Seattle, Washington, have shown that about 25% of people don't need aspirin because their platelets aren't sticky. The other 75% of people have sticky platelets. About 2/3 of these people have platelets that respond adequately to aspirin and 1/3 do not.

The only way to find out who needs treatment to control excessive platelet aggregation and with what medication is to *do appropriate tests.* **The Hope Heart Institute**'s staff is developing and evaluating such tests.

3. Select a Good Doctor and Follow His or Her Advice

If your physician finds that you have a "gene" problem (very high blood level of LDL cholesterol with a family or personal history of heart disease at the young age of 35 to 40 years), he or she may advise either the Pritikin or the Ornish diet for you. These diets limit calories from all types of fat to not over 10% of the total (see p. 3 for our preference).

If you retain fluid, your physician will request that you restrict your salt intake. Also, this may be necessary if you have high blood pressure. It's easy to take too much salt since about 90% of what we ingest is already in the packaged, canned, and fast foods we eat. Read the labels.

Your physician may find that you need medications to decrease your blood pressure and lower your blood levels of LDL cholesterol, triglycerides, glucose, and homocysteine, and to raise your blood levels of HDL cholesterol and omega-3 fatty acids. The highest sources of these essential fatty acids are flaxseed and fish oils (pp. 10,26,67).

You may need *magnesium* since most people are deficient in this essential mineral that steadies and strengthens the heart beat and decreases high blood pressure.

If you are a woman who has passed through menopause, your physician may advise you to take estrogen to reduce your risk of developing coronary heart disease, osteoporosis, and possibly Alzheimer's disease.

While medications are *not* a substitute for the five cardinal rules and the three additional strategies for healthy living, they can be very important.

Section V:
Glossary

Atherosclerosis (Hardening of the Arteries/Arteriosclerosis) - Disease of epidemic proportions in developed nations where it causes more deaths than all types of cancer, accidents, and infections combined. It is due in large measure to smoking; obtaining too many calories from low-fiber carbohydrates, refined sugar, saturated fats, and *trans* fatty acids; leading a sedentary life; gaining excess weight (fat); and letting stress control and distort our lives.

In most patients, this disease causes the inner portion of the arterial wall to become thick, inelastic, and hardened due to plaques formed by infiltration of LDL cholesterol, other fats, and variable amounts of calcium from the blood. Plaques with lots of calcification are hard and those with little are soft. Many soft plaques develop a central collection (core) of thick, slimy, fatty fluid that is covered over by a thin cap of fibrous tissue. If the cap ruptures, this deadly, syrupy liquid in the core oozes into the flow channel where it can trigger the platelets to form clots. Such clots are the most common cause of heart attacks.

Atherosclerosis often makes the arterial flow surface lose its delicate lining of endothelial cells as the inner wall becomes rough, irregular, and ulcerated. If the blood flow slows or becomes turbulent, the diseased flow surface may cause clots to form which block the channel and stop the flow of blood. Whether by this process or by rupture of a soft plaque with a lipid core, the flow channel can become blocked by clot and cause heart attacks, strokes, high blood pressure (hypertension), kidney failure, decreased walking capacity, and amputations.

In a lesser number of patients, the atherosclerotic process weakens the arterial wall so much, most commonly of the aorta in the abdomen, that the blood pressure forces the wall to bulge out and form enlargements called aneurysms, which may rupture and cause fatal hemorrhage.

There is a current suspicion, still unproven, that the bacterium, *Chlamydia pneumoniae,* as well as some viruses, may infect the arterial wall and be part of the "hardened" artery problem. The question of which comes first, like the chicken or the egg, will be the subject of much future research.

Carbohydrates (plant foods - Fiber, also see pp. 68,69) - Organic compounds constructed of carbon, hydrogen, and oxygen, usually in a ratio of 1:2:1. Most of these compounds are polysaccharides which are called complex carbohydrates. They are broken down in the intestines by the digestive enzymes into the monosaccharide glucose ($C_6H_{12}O_6$) -- a simple sugar -- which is absorbed into the blood and carried to the cells where it is used to produce energy. Sucrose ($C_{12}H_{22}O_{11}$) -- table sugar (processed from sugar cane and sugar beets) -- is a non-fiber disaccharide which is quickly broken down into glucose and fructose by the addition of water ("hydrolysis"). Fructose is converted into glucose in the liver. The brain cells and the cells of the retina can only use glucose for energy; other cells can also use fatty acids.

Excess glucose in plants and animals is stored in the same form ($C_6H_{10}O_5$)x, called starch in plants and *glycogen* in animals. *Insulin,* a hormone secreted by the pancreas, in reponse to increased levels of glucose in the blood, enables the cells to use glucose for energy and converts the excess glucose into glycogen, which is stored 1/3 in the liver and 2/3 in muscles. A bit less than a pound of glycogen can be stored in the entire body. Above this level, glucose is rapidly converted into saturated fat and stored in the fat cells of the adipose tissue throughout the body. High levels of insulin block the use of fat for energy. When glucose levels fall due to fasting or exercise, a rise in *glucagon,* another hormone secreted by the pancreas, converts glycogen back into glucose. When all the glycogen is used up, blood glucose falls and insulin levels decrease. This allows fat to be used for energy.

Cholesterol - A fat-like substance ($C_{25}H_{47}OH$) used by the body in making the retaining walls of all cells, the male and female sex hormones, and the hormones secreted by the outer part (the cortex) of the adrenal gland which controls vital chemistry of stress, minerals, sugar, and water.

Cholesterol is transported in the blood in one of three forms, high density lipoprotein cholesterol (HDL), low density lipoprotein cholesterol (LDL), and very low density lipoprotein cholesterol (VLDL). The high concentrations of LDL, low concentrations of HDL, and high levels of triglycerides which are found in VLDL all predispose to the development of atherosclerosis. VLDL and LDL favor atherosclerosis by increasing delivery of cholesterol into the inner portion of the arterial wall. HDL protects against atherosclerosis by transporting LDL cholesterol to the liver which excretes it in the bile. This lowers the blood level of LDL cholesterol and removes some LDL from the arterial wall as well.

Saturated fats and *trans* fatty acids raise LDL cholesterol levels in the blood primarily because they block the receptors for LDL in the liver and in other cells. Excesses of carbohydrates and proteins also raise LDL levels because they are converted into saturated fat which blocks more receptors.

In general, LDL cholesterol begins to infiltrate the inner wall of our arteries when the blood level rises above 130mg/dL. This is the reason why it's so important to: (1) keep our weight under control; and (2) not allow the calories from saturated fats and *trans* fatty acids in our diet to exceed 10% of the total calories we consume in a day. Calorie wise, a little fat goes a long way. LDL cholesterol is bad only if it gets too high. It's a little like water. We can die of dehydration if we don't have enough, but we can drown in it if we have too much. We need the right amount. LDL cholesterol is the same. Below 100 mg/dL is best

Coronary Heart Disease Due to Atherosclerosis - A condition in which there is an insufficient supply of oxygenated (red) blood to the heart muscle because the coronary arteries have become narrowed or even closed off as a result of hardening and thickening of their walls and clot formation on their flow surfaces (coronary thrombosis). This clotting occurs most often as a consequence of rupture of the lipid core of soft plaques which releases its fatty contents into the lumen and causes the blood to jell, i.e., clot. If the artery clots off suddenly, the person may "drop dead."

Clotting also occurs from platelet aggregation and fibrin formation on rough and irregular atherosclerotic surfaces that have lost their covering of endothelial cells.

People with coronary disease often experience pain in the left side of the front of their chest during/after exercise or exertion. If you have this symptom (angina) see your doctor promptly.

Diabetes - A condition characterized by high blood sugar, high urine production, and inability of the cells to use glucose due to lack of, or insensitivity to, insulin, a hormone secreted by the beta cells of the islets of the pancreas. Obesity predisposes to the onset of diabetes in adults. Diabetes predisposes to blindness, kidney failure, and atherosclerosis.

Emphysema - A condition mainly caused by smoking which destroys the elastic tissue of the lungs, causing the patient to slowly suffocate.

Fats (Triglycerides) - Molecules that consist of three fatty acids chemically linked to a three-carbon chain alcohol called glycerol. All fats contain mixtures of different types of fatty acids. Fatty acids consist of linear chains of carbon atoms with hydrogen atoms bound to them. Ninety-five percent of the fat stored in the fat cells of the adipose tissue is in the triglyceride form. The adipose cells have a huge capacity to store fat.

Fats may be classified as saturated or unsaturated. A saturated fatty acid has no double carbon=carbon bonds; all of the bonding sites are filled with hydrogen atoms. Unsaturated fatty acids contain one or more double carbon=carbon bonds. If a fatty acid has only one double bond, it is called monounsaturated. If it has two or more, it is polyunsaturated.

Saturated fats, except for coconut and palm oil types, are solids at room temperature, while unsaturated fats (oils) are liquid. Both varieties are insoluble in water. The body uses many fatty acids and can make all but two, alpha linolenic and linoleic, which are polyunsaturated and must be in our diet. Because of this, these are "essential." Linoleic acid has a double bond between carbons 6 and 7 (omega-6). Alpha linolenic acid has a double bond between carbons 3 and 4 (omega-3). The ideal ratio of omega-6 to omega-3 fatty acids is about 4:1, or even lower. In the average American's diet, the ratio is much higher, being an unfavorable 20:1 or even worse.

Each fat or oil is a unique combination of saturated, monounsaturated, and polyunsaturated omega-6 (linoleic) and omega-3 (alpha linolenic) fatty acids. Olive, canola, avocado, and peanut oils are primarily monounsaturated and are protective against atherosclerosis. Oils containing omega-3 fatty acids (ranked in order of most to least) are:

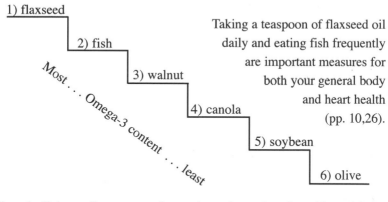

1) flaxseed
2) fish
3) walnut
4) canola
5) soybean
6) olive

Most . . . Omega-3 content . . . least

Taking a teaspoon of flaxseed oil daily and eating fish frequently are important measures for both your general body and heart health (pp. 10,26).

Though all these oils are protective against atherosclerosis and harmful clot formation, flaxseed and fish oils are most protective.

Diets high in saturated fats and *trans* fatty acids increase the blood level of low density lipoprotein cholesterol (LDL). This is so because the saturated fats and *trans* fatty acids reduce the activity of the LDL receptors which is the main mechanism whereby LDL cholesterol is removed from the blood stream by the cells of the body, primarily by those in the liver.

Prime sources of saturated fats are fatty meats, unskinned poultry (skin contains nearly all the fat), whole milk, cheeses, butter, cream, ice cream, candies, cakes, pies, and most other desserts.

Prime sources of *trans* fatty acids (pp. 4,71) are hydrogenated or partially hydrogenated polyunsaturated vegetable oils. These include treated soybean and canola oils which are used in margarines, especially the hard types, and products such as many types of cookies, crackers, cakes, candies, doughnuts, pies, and other pastries. Hydrogenation adds hydrogen and converts unsaturated liquid fats (oils) into more saturated solid fats. Beware if the content label reads "hydrogenation" to any degree. Recently, the FDA has approved two expensive margarines that have been treated with plant sterols to remove most of the *trans* fatty acids from these products. But more research is needed to establish their true worth.

Phospholipids, a special type of fat that contains phosphorus, is the main building material for the walls of the 100 trillion cells that make up our body. If these membranes were to dissolve in water, we would die in seconds. From this aspect alone, fat is an essential part of our diet and body. In addition, our brain is 60% fat. But, we must be selective in what fats we eat. Saturated fats and *trans* fatty acids types can damage our arteries and must be severely restricted.

Protective (unsaturated) fats (see p. 67) are not only good for us, they add taste and satisfaction to our meals. But they are such a rich source of calories (9 calories/gram) that they must be eaten in moderation to maintain balance in our diet. If we don't eat for 12 to 18 hours or run for many miles, our main source of energy shifts from glucose to fatty acids as our meager stores of glycogen (storage from of glucose) are quickly used up (p. 65).

Fiber - The portion of plant (carbohydrate) foods that our bodies can't digest. There are two basic types of fiber -- soluble and insoluble. Insoluble fiber helps the digestive system run smoothly and prevents constipation. Soluble fiber decreases the absorption of cholesterol by the intestines.

Insoluble fiber ("roughage") includes the woody parts of plants, such as the skins of fruits and vegetables and the outer coating of grain and rice kernels.

Soluble fiber dissolves and thickens in water to form gels. Beans, barley, broccoli, citrus fruits, oatmeal, and especially oat bran are rich sources of soluble fiber.

Fiber is found only in complex carbohydrates. Whether the fiber is soluble or insoluble, complex carbohydrates that are coated by their natural protective fiber components are digested and absorbed more slowly than when the fiber has been removed by refining processes. A high-fiber content slows the digestion of complex carbohydrates and decreases the glucose load on the islet cells of the pancreas. This lowers the demand for insulin and reduces the tendency to develop adult-onset diabetes.

This is why the majority of our carbohydrate calories should come from high-fiber sources, such as fresh fruits; fresh vegetables; and legumes (peas, beans, and lentils); whole-grain breads, cereals, and pastas; and whole grains, such as brown rice. **The Better Life Diet** is high-fiber.

This is also why we should markedly restrict the calories we get from low-fiber processed complex carbohydrates (such as white bread, mashed potatoes, french fries -- also have too much fat -- and white rice) because they have lost most of their fiber. Refined sugar (mainly sucrose), a totally non-fiber, disaccharide carbohydrate, $(C_{12}H_{22}O_{11})$, is quickly combined in the intestines with water and converted into glucose and fructose (both $C_6H_{12}O_6$ monosaccharides) more rapidly than occurs even with the low-fiber foods. For this reason, refined sugar should be drastically restricted in our diet because it is harmful to our health.

Fiber is also valuable because it contains many minerals, phytochemicals (plant chemicals), and vitamins.

Heart Attack - A condition in which part of the heart muscle dies because of lack of blood supply, most often due to from obstruction (occlusion) of a coronary artery due to atherosclerosis and clot formation (thrombosis). The impact of a heart attack may be mild, moderate, severe, or even fatal depending on how much and which part of the heart muscle has lost its blood supply. The patient suffering a heart attack will often experience severe chest pain, become nauseated, sweat profusely, develop marked shortness of breath, have low blood pressure, and feel very weak.

Insulin - A hormone secreted by the beta cells of the islets of the pancreas in response to the level of glucose in blood. Insulin enables all the cells of the body to use glucose for energy, converts extra glucose into glycogen for storage in the liver and muscles, and stops the use of fat for energy (p.65).

Osteoporosis A disorder in which bone structure is absorbed. This weakens the skeleton, shortens its stature, and predisposes the bones to fractures, especially of the hip and spine.

Platelets - Tiny pinched off portions of a large cell in the bone marrow called a *megakaryocyte*. These fragments float along in the outer portion of the blood stream ever ready to initiate formation of a clot to plug up holes in the blood vessel walls. Platelets can also form harmful clots (p.64).

Besides being fundamental in the process of clot formation, platelets contain many growth factors that promote the healing of wounds. Platelets survive 10 days after they are released into the blood from the bone marrow. Each second 1-1/2 million platelets wear out and are replaced by 1-1/2 million new ones. While too few platelets can cause us to bleed to death, too many can cause us to clot to death.

Proteins - Complex, big molecules constructed of long, three-dimensionally wrapped chains of combinations of amino acids. Amino acids are molecules constructed of four chemical units joined to a single carbon atom: an amino (NH_2) group, a hydrogen atom (H), a carboxylic acid (COOH) group, and a side-group containing various combinations of carbon, hydrogen, nitrogen (N), and sometimes sulfur (S). Side-groups distinguish the 20 different amino acids that our bodies must have.

Of these 20 amino acids, nine can't be manufactured by our bodies and must be derived from the foods we eat. These amino acids, which we must have but can't manufacture, are called *essential* amino acids.

The body manufactures thousands of different types of proteins from different combinations of these 20 amino acids. Each of these proteins has a single function. This function is determined by the order and shape of its amino acid chains.

Many vital structures inside our cells are made from proteins. For example, the ribosomes that make proteins and the mitochondria that make energy are constructed with proteins. The enzymes that control the chemistry of our bodies are also proteins. The hemoglobin in our red blood cells that carries the oxygen upon which our lives depend is a protein. Our muscles are proteins. The external surface features of our bodies (eyes, ears, nose, skin, hair, and nails) are made of proteins.

As discussed previously, obesity can lead to many serious medical problems. On the other hand, being very thin is also very dangerous. If people who are very thin can't eat for some reason, their depleted muscles are progressively consumed for energy since they have no remaining glycogen or fat stores to sustain them.

Clearly, proteins are essential for life. Also, they provide taste and satisfaction to our meals. Proteins are best obtained from fish, skinless poultry, eggs, peas, beans, lentils, nuts, seeds, nonfat/low-fat dairy products, and low-fat meat, such as lean beef, lamb, and center cut pork loin/chop or roast.

Risk Factors - Conditions that predispose to the development of a certain disease. For example, risk factors for having a heart attack include:

- Smoking.
- Eating a low-fiber diet high in refined sugar, saturated fats, *trans* fatty acids, and calories.
- Leading a sedentary life.
- Carrying significant excess weight (fat).
- Experiencing marked stress.
- Having a family history of heart disease.
- Possessing sticky platelets, high fibrinogen, low HDL cholesterol, high LDL cholesterol, high triglycerides, and/or elevated levels of homocysteine.
- Having high blood pressure, diabetes, gout, and/or low thyroid function.

Sugar (Sucrose - $C_{12}H_{22}O_{11,}$ pp. 64,65) - a non-fiber disaccharide (carbohydrate) with a sweet taste that is refined in crystalline or powdered form from sugar cane or sugar beets for use in foods to improve taste.

Syndrome X - Condition affecting a growing number of people identified by the chemical triad of low HDL cholesterol, high triglycerides, and a decreased sensitivity to high blood levels of insulin. This triad is associated with a strong tendency to develop obesity, hypertension, and adult-onset diabetes. The **Better Life Diet** and **Exercise Program** is ideal to correct this chemical disorder.

Trans **Fatty Acids (Fats)** - an altered form of vegetable oils produced by the process of hydrogenation which addds hydrogen atoms to the unsaturated carbon chains which converts these liquid oils into soft solids at room temperature. These hydrogenated chains resemble those of saturated fats and are called *trans* fatty acids. Examples of such changes are found in the conversion of soybean and canola oils into soft solids in the manufacture of margarines, and of peanut oil in the manufacture of peanut butter. These altered oils are even more dangerous to your heart than saturated fats.

Index

Alcohol, 16

Antioxidants, 61

Aspirin, 62

Atherosclerosis, 8,55,62,64

Better Life Diet, 1-3,5-9,11,14-26,55-59,60

Carbohydrates, 1-3,5-9,65,68,69

Cholesterol, 2-4,56,57,60,63,65,66

Coronary Heart Disease due to atherosclerosis, 2,3,55,66

Diabetes (adult-onset), 3,8,15,66

Dietary Goals (7) of Better Life Diet, 5

Emphysema, 66

Exercise, 3,5,27-53

Fats (Triglycerides), 2-9,11-16,66-68,71

Fiber, 1,2,7-9,58,59,68,69

Fibrinogen, 57,60

Five Cardinal Rules for Healthy Living, 54-58

Flaxseed oil, 3,10,26,63,67

Food Guide Diagram, 6

Glossary, 64-71

HDL Cholesterol, 60,65,66

Healthy Living

    Five Cardinal Rules, 54-58

    Simple Plan, 54-63

    Three Additional Strategies, 60-63

Heart Attack, 2,3,55,69

High Blood Pressure (hypertension), 3,55

Homocysteine, 56,60,61

Insulin, 3,7,8,14,16,65,69

LDL Cholesterol, 2,56,57,60,61,65,66

Magnesium, 63

Meal Plan (7 day) and Nurtitional Analysis for Better Life Diet©, 17-26

Milk, classification, 7

Nutritional Basis for Better Life Diet© and Weight Control, 1-16

Obesity, 2,3,9,15,66

Omega-3 & -6 essential fatty acids, 10,26,63,67

Ornish diet, 63

Osteoporosis, 28,69

Plaque, 55,64

Platelet Aggregation, 69,70

Platelets, 62,70

Prevention of Atherosclerosis (hardening of the arteries)

    Dietary Information, 1-16

    Exercise, 27-53

    Simple Plan for Healthy Living, 54-63

    Smoking, 55-58

    Stress, 55-58

    Weight, 14-16,55-58

Pritikin diet, 63

Proteins, 1-3,5-7,57,58,70,71

Risk Factors for Heart Attack, 71

Simple Plan for Healthy Living, 54-63

Smoking, 55-58

Stress, 55-58

Stroke, 2,55

Sugar, 1-3,7-9,14-16,57-60,63,71

Syndrome X, 14,71

Trans Fatty Acids, 1-5,7-9,13,57,59,71

Triglycerides (Fats), 1-9,11-16,66-68,71

Weight - How to - -

    lose excess, 14-16

    gain when too thin, 16

    maintain stable status, 16

Special Notes

One day in November, 1999, I had a call from **Tom DeBuys** of Seattle who had read my book, *The Open Heart*. He asked me to sign it for him, which I was happy to do. We started chatting, and I was soon very impressed with all the research into diet that he had done. So, I asked him to read the nutrition section from my nearly finished book, *The Better Life Diet*.

Though Tom is a busy lawyer, he soon started working with me in a nonstop, enthusiastic manner on how I could communicate information to the layperson in an even better way.

For that immeasurable help, I express my deepest thanks to Tom for making the *Better Life Diet: A Simple Plan for a Long and Youthful Life* a more effective means to bring life-saving information in an easily understood manner to people around the world.

Other Books by Lester R. Sauvage, MD

The Open Heart: Secret to Happiness - Forewords by Mother Teresa and C. Everett Koop. Dr. Sauvage and ten of his patients tell you from the depths of their souls what matters most in life and how to find it.

You Can Beat Heart Disease: Prevention and Treatment - endorsed by 50 of the world's leading medical authorities - easy to understand health information. As Dr. David Robinson of the NIH said: "All Americans should read this book."

For further information call Better Life Press at 206/323-0116, or visit . . . http://www.drsauvage.com. If you are a book retailer or other book seller, please contact **Independent Publishers Group**, 814 N. Franklin Street, Chicago, Illinois, U.S.A. 60610. Phone: 800/888-4741 or 312/337-0747.